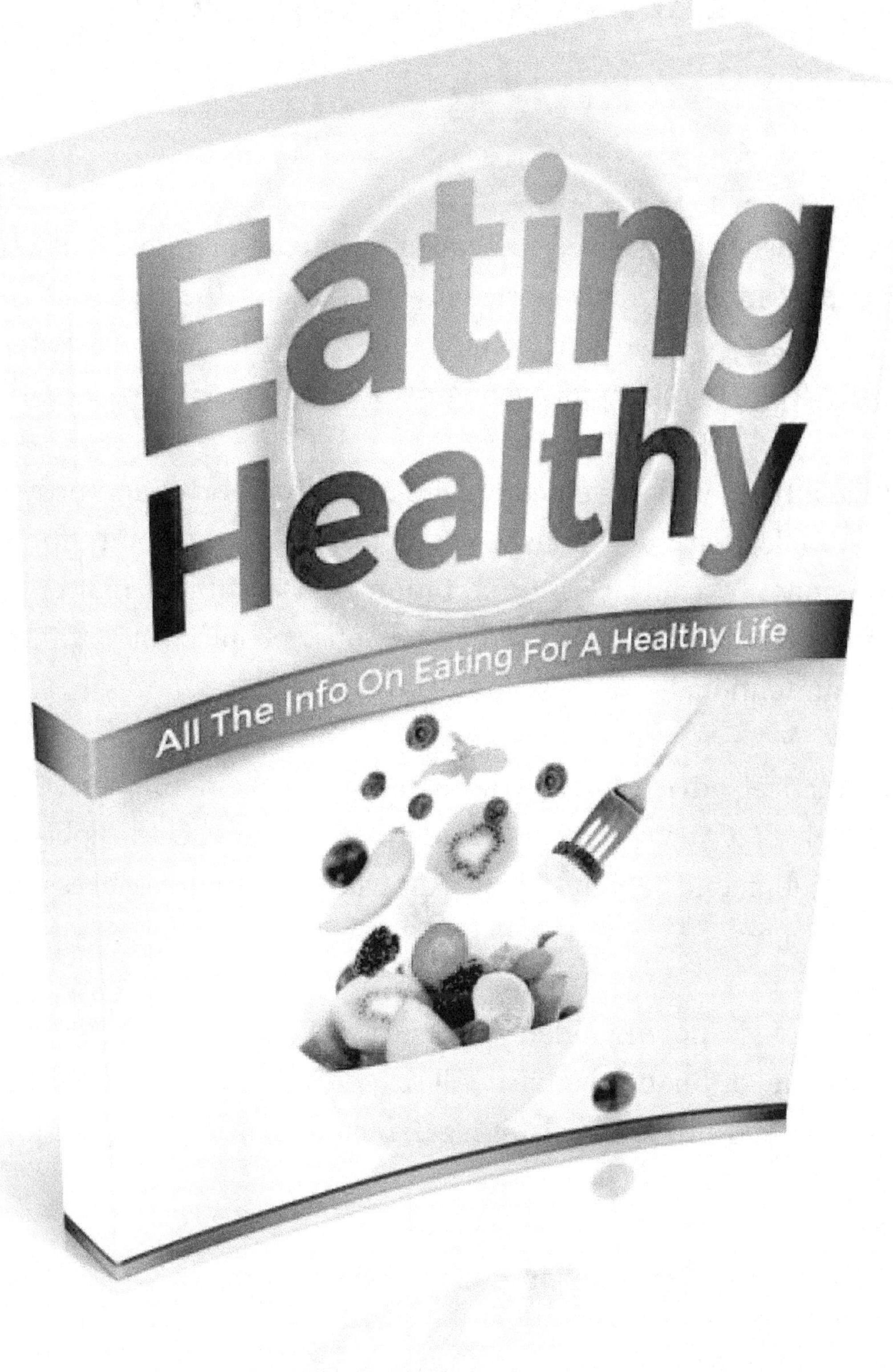

Eating Healthy

All The Info On Eating For A Healthy Life

Terms and Conditions

LEGAL NOTICE

Table Of Contents

Foreword

In simple terms the body has two very different and complex systems of energy producing sources. As energy is vital to the very existence of human activity and survival the two energy style depend on each other for support. This book shows you what foods give you the most energy.

It occurs so very frequently - we resolve to go on with a health and physical fitness program with zest and likely much fanfare too; however in the first week of going into the plan, everything peters out.

Why is it that we don't stick with the diet plans, the morning jogging plans, the physical exercise plans that we make?

And what may we do to ensure we keep going with these plans, for our own sake and for the sake of the individuals that are dependent on us?

Are you eating simply to satisfy your appetite or to make your taste buds happy? Or are you eating in order to take better command of your life? In this eBook, we see how you are able to make your life much more optimal simply by making a point that you eat correctly.

Eating Healthy
All The Info On Eating For A Healthy Life

Chapter 1:

The Basics

Synopsis

Energy is needed for the various functions like maintenance of growth, daily activities, exercise and many other movements or functions that are often taken for granted. These are shared between the two energy systems.

In today's world, seldom do any health and fitness plans work. What's the reason for their alarming rate of failure?

The world is a lot less healthful than it was two decades ago. Much this is attributed to the altered food habits of individuals.

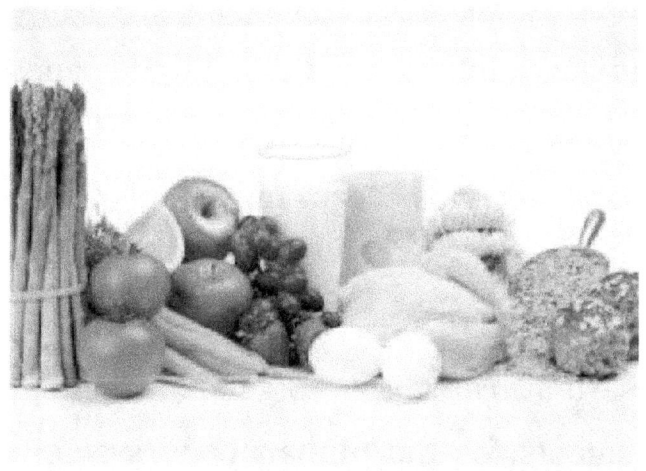

The Basics

The primary and first to be used energy system is the aerobic system. This system uses oxygen for the function of the muscles and does demand quite a lot from the general body system.

This demand usually increases the rate and depth of breathing and blood supply mainly because of the corresponding increase of the heart rate.

When the body requires more energy which cannot be met due to the elevated need for more oxygen then the body system automatically switched to the anaerobic energy system. This system is able to produce energy without the need to use oxygen.

All this energy is generated through the suitable or correct consumption of foods. The foods consumed dictate the types of energy levels each individual is capable of producing.

Muscle fatigue usually occurs when all the energy sources are exhausted which can be attributed to a variety of reasons; the most compelling one depends very much on the types of foods consumed.

There are several categories of foods that produce various beneficial elements for the human body system and noting the ones that create or enhance the energy generating sources is definitely useful to know. Therefore this knowledge should help the individual choose the right types of foods.

The aerobic system works by breaking down the carbohydrates, fatty acids and amino acids in the foods consumed while the anaerobic system releases energy from the foods stored in the body, usually during intense activity bouts.

If we hear about the failure of diets or gym plans all around us, commonly it isn't their fault. Commonly it is the fault of the individuals who started with much commotion about going through these plans, telling all their acquaintances and co-workers about it, and then didn't abide by those programs.

The individuals who abandon the exercise or diet halfway do not see the advantages, naturally, and everybody blames the plan.

What the world needs nowadays isn't a fresh health or fitness program or a diet, but it requires motivation. It needs the correct sort of mind-set to follow through with whatever plan they have chosen to the very end.

If they can do that, most of the health issues that are related to life-style situations will get to be outmoded. And we don't have to visit the corners of the earth to discover this motivation. The motivation lies right here, inside us; we simply need to search it out and utilize it.

One generation ago, individuals wouldn't dream of picking up whatever junk food they could get in order to feed their faces. Nowadays, we do that so very casually. "I'm hungry" commonly means "I want a burger or a hot dog, likely with chips on the side and some cola." And, "I am on a diet" means "I am on a chemically ridden pill which will defeat my hunger and deprive my body of vitamins." It's genuinely no wonder that we are facing so many health issues today.

Our health is an indicator of what we consume. The sorry condition that we're living in isn't an individual problem; it's a global issue. The world as a whole is eating incorrectly. Six in every ten individuals in the US is overweight, and the number is going to be eight in every ten individuals by the time we hit 2015.

Are we truly thinking about this? We aren't. Even as you're studying this eBook, you likely have a packet of chips on the side. Do you know that what you spent on that package, which is filling your stomach with some of the most toxic chemicals known to humanity, could instead have fed an emaciated youngster in Ruanda?

But it's not simply about being philanthropic. It's about ourselves too. Yes, we have to be selfish. With such appalling health figures, aren't we heading for doom? We're definitely not eating right. Whatever excess baggage that brings - obesity and the assorted ill health in its wake - we have to be prepared for it.

So the next time you see that a program has failed or is receiving a lot of criticism, remember that the criticism isn't probably because the program stands on shaky ground. In most cases, it is because people began with great intentions and then did not follow the program as they should have

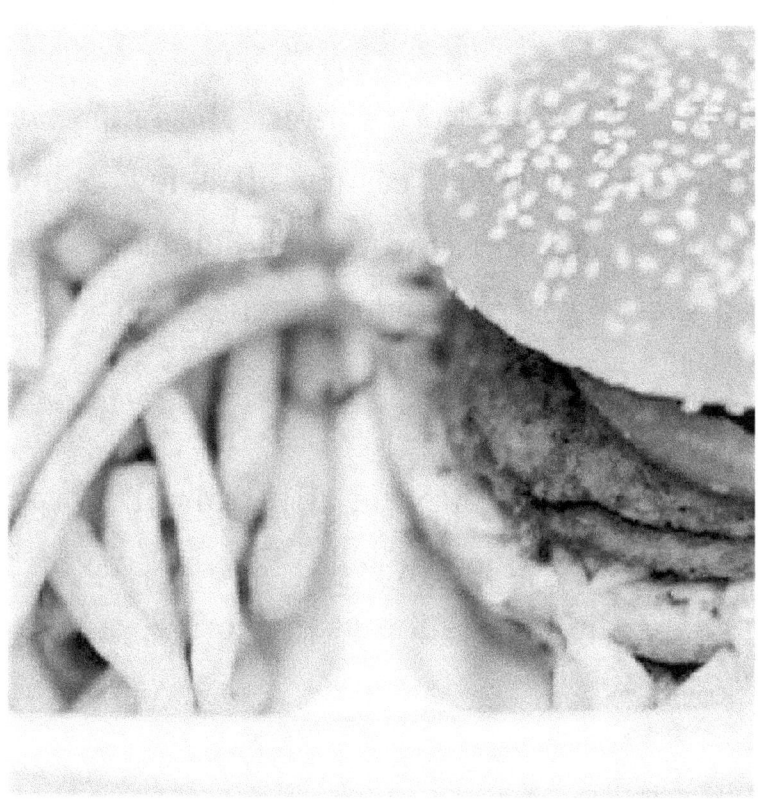

Chapter 2:

The Way You Think About Food

Synopsis

The most crucial thing that you need to keep your health and fitness program alive - even more crucial than an instructor or a doctor - is your own motive.

You have to be determined to scrutinize the situation. So, you're overweight and are looking at casting off a few pounds. No gym instructor from anyplace in the world will help you if you don't take adequate measures to have the right diet and to stick to your routine exercise.

Even if you're sick and are looking at treatment, no physician will help if you aren't determined in following the treatment platform, whether it's taking the medication at the correct time or abstaining from some foods.

Your Mindset

We have strayed horribly with our eating habits thus far. Unless we take stock of the state of affairs and take matters in our own hands, matters are not going to get better.

The number 1 thing is awareness. We have to learn what foods are correct for us and what are not. We have to go back to training and comprehend what the nutrients are that your body truly wants and in what amount.

Then we have to build a dietary regimen for ourselves and our loved ones so that we eat healthier. We have to cut down on all the foods that are adverse - the sugars, the fats, the carbohydrates, we don't truly want them - and incorporate foods that may boost our health.

This does sound too preachy, I understand. But that's the only reprieve we have got. If we continue munching on Oreos, we're never going to get better.

But there's hope. Hope lies in the fact that there are a lot of foods out there that are simply as tasty as those awful junk foods but we don't yet know about them.

These are the foods that we don't know about yet, we likely don't care for them or as we don't know how to fix them, but a healthy cookbook may help you in understanding assorted interesting ways to healthy cooking.

Even with the same sort of diet you eat, you are able to conjure up some really delicious healthy dishes. Yes, it's all very much possible. You are able to modify your eating habits to a big extent, while at the same time attending to your palate.

The fact is that the weight loss industry is responsible in a really significant way towards this downfall of the developed human race. They have to keep selling their Atkinses and Jenny Craigs and Zones and Medifasts and for that reason the media never tells you how we may in reality take things in your own hands.

They show us glitzy before-after pictures of a person with a foot-long sub and then the same guy with 6 pack abs and tell us that the diet made that possible.

However the fact is, if we were to get our head together, we may very easily do that too, without having to spend 1000s of dollars on those diets. And what do we have to do?

<u>2 general things:-</u>

Control what we consume.
Indulge in physical exertion.

Now, is that too much to accomplish? Don't we owe that to our body that has served us so well all these years? Don't we owe that to ourselves and our loved ones?

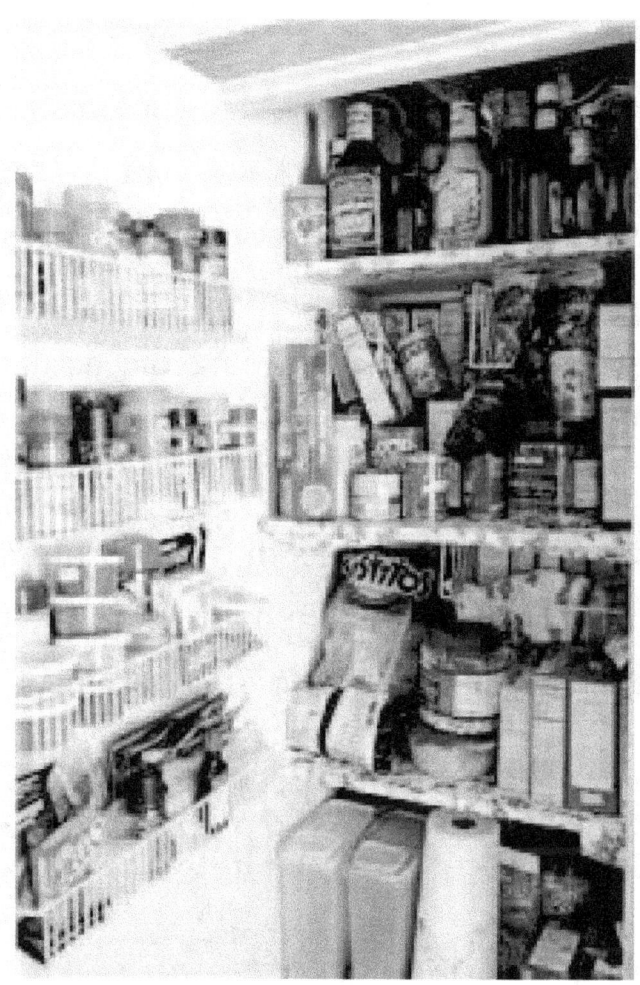

Chapter 3:

Honey And Whole Grains

Synopsis

Over the years honey has been proven to the one sustaining power behind the energy circle. Benefiting the human body in various areas it is foremost still unrivaled in its energy producing entity. Honey is nature's most natural energy booster. It also acts as an effective immunity system builder while providing the natural remedy to a host of varied ailments too.

Energy is very important to the smooth flowing natural of a daily life cycle of any human being. Therefore finding energy sources that are both consistent and healthy are important to keeping fit and happy.

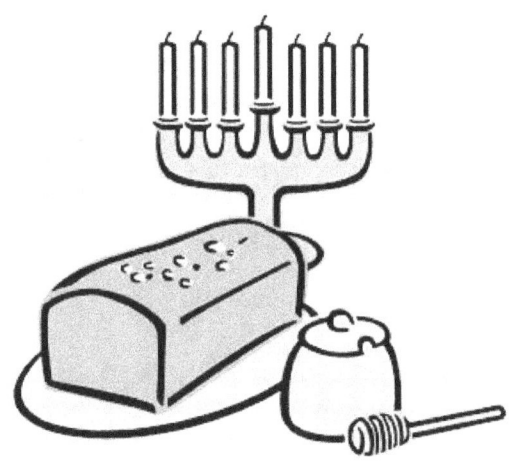

A Good Pair

The natural benefits of honey has been widely acknowledged and accepted. Besides its great taste, honey is also a natural source of carbohydrate, which is an energy maker for boosting performance, endurance and reducing levels of muscle fatigue.

This is especially useful for athletes. The sugar content in the honey helps to play a role in preventing fatigue during exercise sessions and also during training sessions for sports enthusiast. These sugar make ups are divided into glucose and fructose and functions in different but complimenting ways.

The glucose content in the honey is generally absorbed at a faster rate and gives off an immediate energy boost while the fructose works at a slower pace for a more sustainable and prolonged energy dispersement. When it comes to addressing blood sugar levels in the body system, honey has been known to help keep the levels fairly constant.

As honey is a pleasant food product and it's natural in its form, consuming it is not a very difficult exercise. People of all ages are generally quite willing to consume honey in any of its accompanying forms. It's even popular with children.

The energy produced from consuming a small amount of honey daily helps children cope with the physical strains of daily school activities and sports commitments. For the adults too consuming a daily small dose of honey can go a long way in keeping the energy levels at its best during a demanding day at work.

Making sandwiches with honey accompanied with other fillings is one way of creating a pleasant snack. Applying honey on a freshly toasted slice of bread is also a welcome breakfast alternative. Adding honey to drinks instead of using sugar is definitely encouraged.

Most people today want a quick fix for their energy boosting needs and this usually comes in the unhealthy forms of sports drinks, coffee and refined carbohydrates like sugar and while bread.

Though these produce the desired heightened energy levels, it should be noted that this energy is fairly short lived and the tiredness that follows is usually more acutely felt. Therefore opting to consume some form of whole grains is not only a better alternative but is also much healthier.

Whole grains provide the energy that comes in a more complex form which breaks down over a longer period of time. This then creates the platform for sustaining the energy levels for longer periods.

Because of its more complex make up the whole grains come with a array of beneficial elements like minerals, vitamins, phytonutrients and fiber which are also rich in fiber.

Adding the whole grain ingredients is any dish more often than not completes the flavor or enhances it altogether. Whole grains can the various forms such as wheat, oat, barley, maize, brown rice, faro, spelt, emmer, einkorn, rye, millet, buckwheat, and many more.

These can then be made into various other products like whole wheat flour, whole wheat bread, whole wheat pasta, rolled oats or oat groats, triticale flour, popcorn and teff flour.

The benefits of consuming whole grains consistently can help decrease the risk of heart disease, lower cholesterol levels protect against many types of cancer and assist in weight management. Whole grains should not be confused with its lesser and more refined "cousin". Though refined grains have some benefits it is always better to opt for the whole grain alternatives

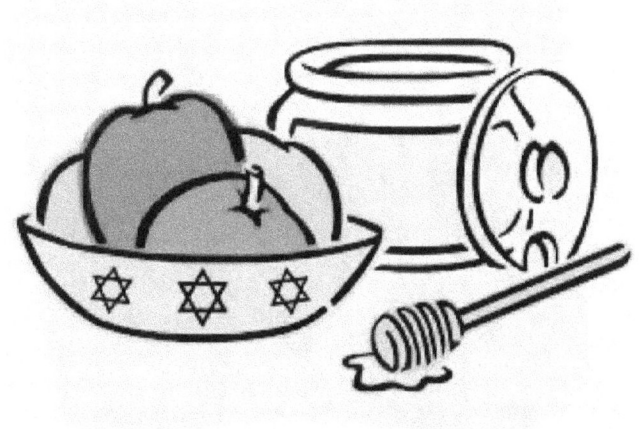

Chapter 4:

Nuts And Lean Meat

Synopsis

Nuts are an important source of nutrients for both human and animal consumption. Being rich in a whole host of necessary nutrients it can be eaten in its raw form, cooked or as an additive to already pre existing dishes. Thought nuts are defined as a hard shelled fruit, there are many other foods that are included in the nut family.

Different types of meats generally contribute to a variety of flavors; however the healthiest type is the one with as much lean meat content as possible. Its undisputed fact that the meats that contain a good amount of fat are a culinary treat indeed but for health purposes taking the time to understand the benefits of consuming lean meats is very wise indeed.

Good Proteins And Oils

It is now common knowledge that nuts greatly help in keeping a lot of ailments in check or from occurring at all. For instance, nuts have been known to be able to keep the possibility of coronary heart diseases manifesting, even for those whole come from a long line of family members with this problem.

Consuming nuts like almonds and walnuts have been known to lower serum cholesterol concentrations within the body system. Nuts are also highly recommended for those individuals suffering from insulin resistance problems like diabetics.

Turning to nuts rather that junk food to quell cravings is also another healthier alternative. Containing essential fatty acids is also another plus point when it comes to choosing nuts as a healthier alternative. Because nuts are healthy and can be consumed in its raw form, it is also another added advantage to keeping these around and handy as snacks.

Almonds are often used to normalize blood lipids because of their slow burn characteristics, which help to keep the blood sugar levels consistently healthy. Rich in a varied amount of different nutrients the almond is a popular additive to the stale diet of most Mediterranean people.

The Brazil nut is also another nutritious nut which comes with its own set of benefits when consumed in moderation. Noted for its omega 3 fatty acid content, the Brazil nut is also a good source of calcium.

Cashew nut is another very popular nut that is often consumed as a salted snack. However it would be a much healthier food product without the addition of salt, as it is already quite a flavorful nut on its own. In some parts of the world these nuts are made into oils.

The selection process should be done with a little knowledge as depending solely on what the naked eye perceives is not enough. Generally lean meats derived from beef cuts should include round, chuck, sirloin and tenderloin, while the cuts from pork or lamb would constitute tenderloin, loin chops and leg. The leanest parts of the poultry would be the breast area without the skin.

Though there are many reasons people eliminate meat from their daily diet, there is no evidence to show that this is a good or bad choice not should it be followed by all.

However the important point to note here is the choice of the types of meats that would make the consumption healthy and this would generally mean meats with lesser amount of fat content. Though white meat is by no means lacking in fat content, it is by comparison much less in fat content than red meats.

The nutritional value of consuming lean meats is quite extensive and rounded. Lean meats have a generally higher and purer content of protein which is a very important contributing factor to fundamental structural and functional progress of every cell sustenance and formation.

Lean meats are also a good source of essential amino acids particularly sulphur amino acids. When compared to the digestive rates the proteins in meats work faster than the one contained in the beans and whole wheat range.

Lean meat is also a good source of iron. Because iron deficiency is progressive it is often not detected until a later stage where anemia has developed.

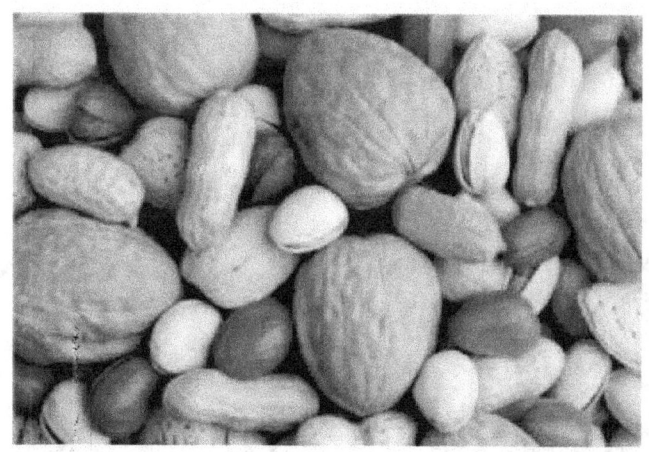

Chapter 5:

The Benefits

Synopsis

Here is all the motive you'd require to continue eating healthy.

Let's immediately plunge into the subject.

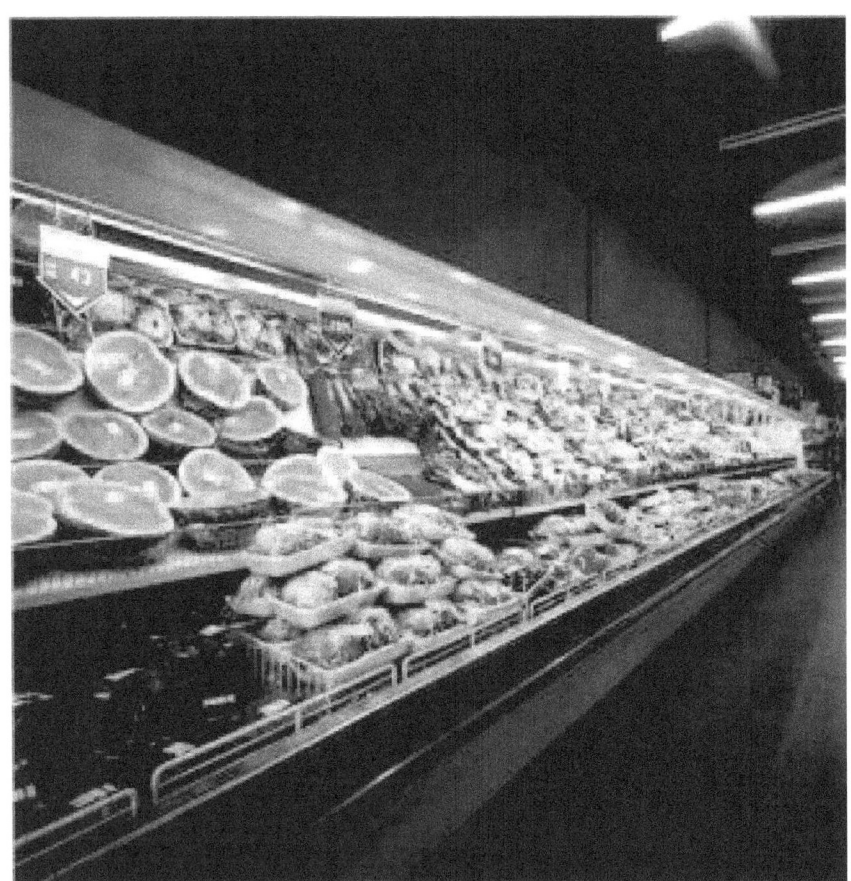

Advantages

You Get Healthier

We might whole collection of books about the health advantages of eating correctly and still it wouldn't quite cover what advantages genuinely exist. The most important advantage is that you gain command over your weight.

By eating correctly, you likewise make certain that your metabolic functions - most notably your immune system and your gastrointestinal system - keep working correctly. You're likewise protected from assorted chronic diseases, right from cardiovascular diseases like coronary artery disease and high blood pressure to diabetes.

More Cost Effective

Eating healthy means you spend much less. Your bills at the supermarkets come down drastically and you don't plunge farther into charge card debt if that is already an issue with you. In addition to that, you save a huge bundle on all the healthcare expenses you'd need if any issue surfaces because of your food binging habits.

Less Toxins In Your Body

A lot of foods nowadays are toxic because of the synthetic chemicals present in them. When you're attempting to eat correctly, you are much less likely to get these toxins into your body as one of the basic dogmas of eating correctly is that you shouldn't eat anything that's man-made.

In addition to that, if you eat less, you'll likewise be able to reduce on vices like smoking and alcoholism. A glass of beer is almost synonymous with a night out with the boys. If you eat less, you won't want the beer as well. Similarly, you will not want that one (or more) mandatory smoke that you tend to have after each meal.

More Physical Lifestyle

When you eat better, you'll find that you are able to do your work in a much better way. You are able to exercise more, travel more, play more, work more and therefore make your life more productive.

That sure beats being a fat slob and lounging around on the couch the whole day, doesn't it? You are able to also be more involved with your friends and loved ones and that surely enriches your life.

Good Social Life

Forget about fat fetishism, individuals who are overweight don't look appealing. There's a strong social taboo about weight on the wrong places of the body. If you're trying to find a partner, your flab may literally get in the way. Not simply that, individuals who can't control their eating habits and hence their weight are looked down upon by society as being individuals who can't control their basic urges.

This sort of psychology does exist, though very few individuals will speak about it. When you eat correctly, you'll discover that such issues disappear.

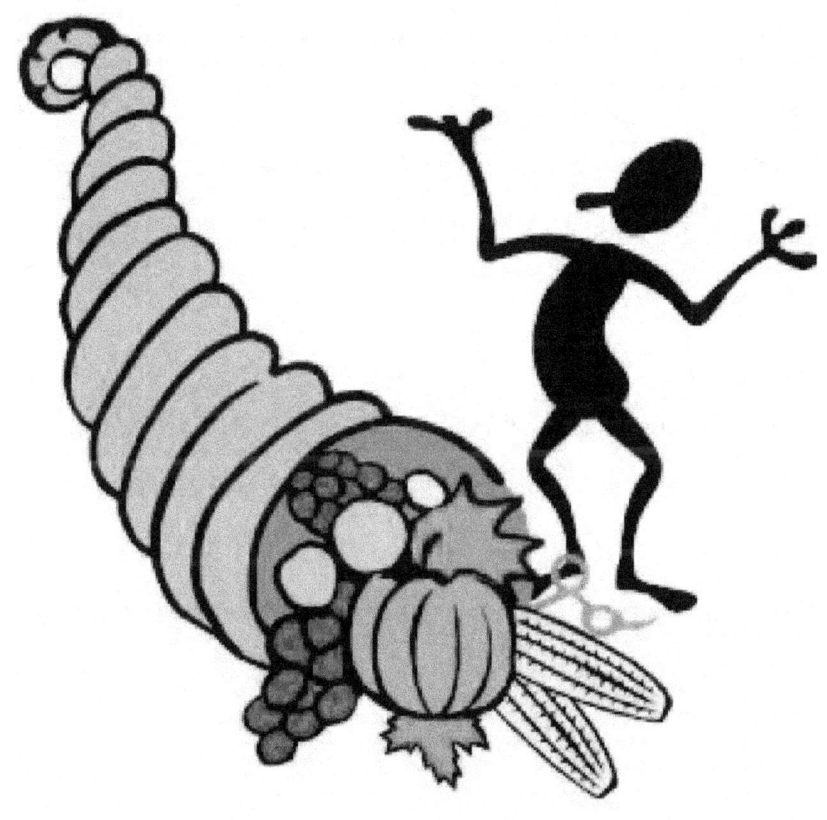

Wrapping Up

There are a lot of popular diets on the market nowadays, but most of them are unhealthy and occasionally even unsafe. This will explain how to eat a healthy, balanced diet for life and keep away from unhealthy diets.

Ascertain how many calories your body requires to function every day.

This number may vary wildly, depending on your metabolism and how physically active you are. If you're the sort of individual who puts on ten pounds simply smelling a slice of pizza, then your every day caloric intake ought to stay approximately 2000 calories for men, and 1500 calories for women.

Your body mass likewise plays a part in that: More calories are appropriate for naturally bigger individuals, and fewer calories for littler individuals. If you're the sort of individual who can eat without gaining a pound, or you're physically active, you might wish to increase your daily caloric intake by 1000-2000 calories, a bit less for women.

Don't dread fatty foods.

You have to consume fat from foods for your body to run correctly. But, it's crucial to pick out the correct sorts of fats: Most animal fats and a few vegetable oils are high in the sort of fats that raise your LDL cholesterol levels; the foul cholesterol.

Different than popular belief, eating cholesterol doesn't inevitably bring up the amount of cholesterol in your body. If you provide your body the correct tools, it will flush extra cholesterol from your body. Those tools are monounsaturated fatty acids, which you ought to try to consume regularly. Foods that are rich in monounsaturated fatty acids are olive oil, nuts, fish oil, and assorted seed oils.

Eat plenty of the correct carbs.

You have to eat foods high in carbs since they're your body's chief source of energy. The trick is to pick out the correct carbs. Simple carbs like sugar and refined flour are quickly absorbed by the body's gastrointestinal system.

This induces a sort of carb overload, and your body releases vast amounts of insulin to battle the overload. Not only is the excess insulin bad on your heart, however it encourages weight gain. Eat plenty of carbs, but consume carbs that are slowly digested by the body such as whole grain flour, veggies, oats, and unprocessed grains.

Eat bigger meals early on in the day.

Your metabolism decelerates toward the end of the evening and is less efficient at digesting foods. That means more of the power stored in the food will be stacked away as fat and your body won't absorb as many nutrients from the meal. Try eating a medium-sized meal for breakfast, a big meal for lunch, and a little meal for dinner. Better yet, attempt consuming 4-6 small meals over the run of your day.

Provide yourself a cheat meal.

Cheating doesn't mean gorging on all the wrong foods once a week; it implies enjoying a food you truly love once a week. Have a couple slices of pizza on Sundays, or a huge slice of double chocolate cake on Saturdays. This cheat meal will help you stick with the change in diet, and in a few ways it's really good for your body. Special occasions, like birthdays in the family, count as cheat meals.

Get the habit of eating slowly.

It will satisfy you with fewer calories and will forestall overeating and obesity with all its consequences.

Drink plenty of H2O.

It makes you feel more awake and energized, does wonders for your skin and makes you feel fuller so you wind up eating less! Cutting down soda and replacing it with water will do wonders for you.